UnBearably Loud

Solutions to Snoring &

Sleep Apnea

by

Bear Lawrence

The information presented is the author's opinion and does not constitute any health or medical advice.

The content of this book is for informational purposes only and is not intended to diagnose, treat, cure, or prevent any condition or disease.

Please seek advice from your healthcare provider for your personal health concerns prior to taking healthcare advice from this book.

I would like to offer my sincere gratitude to

Kevin H. Hilton and Sam Burnell.

Kevin is an author and co-author on the as yet unpublished novel 'Admissions'. He has helped with cover design and worked diligently to both proofread and edit this manuscript.

Sam is an author and my mentor. She has been very kind and generous in sharing her knowledge, experience and time supporting me.

My thanks also to Anastasia Gorskaya who worked with me and my ideas to draw the illustration on the cover of this book.

4

CONTENTS

Foreword and Disclaimer

Part One – My Snoring & My Sleep Apnea Diagnosis

Chapter 1 – Insomnia and Nightmares

Chapter 2 – My Snoring

Chapter 3 – Sleep Study

Part Two - Snoring & Sleep Apnea Explained

Chapter 4 – The Upper Airways

Chapter 5 – Diagnosis

Chapter 6 – Treatments

Chapter 7 – Mandibular Advancement Device

Chapter 8 – CPAP

(CONTENTS continued overleaf)

CONTENTS (continued)

Part Three - Device Experiments

Chapter 9 – Explanation and Experiments

Chapter 10 – Mouthpieces

Chapter 11 – Micro-CPAP

Chapter 12 – Magnetic Nose Clip

Chapter 13 – Nasal Dilators

Chapter 14 – Smart Throat Snorer Stopper

Chapter 15 – Anti-Snoring Chin Strap

Chapter 16 – Anti-Snoring Tongue Device

Part Four - Conclusions

Chapter 17 – Conclusions

Foreword and Disclaimer

Sleep Apnea and Sleep Apnoea are simply different spellings of the same condition. My apologies if you are an 'apnoea' speller as I have used 'apnea' here.

I'm a former university lecturer and we have a mantra for presenting information to students;

'Tell them what you are going to tell them. Tell them. Tell them what you told them.'

I've written several books. I typically use the Foreword for the first part, *'Tell them what you are going to tell them'*. This book is different. Here is my Foreword, which is a Disclaimer:

The information presented is the author's opinion and does not constitute any health or medical advice. The content of this book is for informational purposes only and is not intended to diagnose, treat, cure, or prevent any condition or disease. Please seek advice from your healthcare provider for your personal health concerns prior to taking healthcare advice from this book.

Part One

My Snoring & My Sleep Apnea Diagnosis

Chapter 1 – Insomnia and Nightmares

Even as a child, I never slept well. I found it difficult to sleep and would roam around the house until I incurred the wrath of my parents. On a morning, I'd be up like a lark. I wasn't aware of the word insomnia, or that this was considered a problem, so it never bothered me as a child.

Every so often, my mother would have to wake me up from a nightmare. Sometimes I would be screaming and yet still asleep. Once awake, I would be terrified and it would take a long time for the fear to subside so that I might sleep again.

This pattern of difficulty sleeping and having to be woken whilst screaming having a nightmare, carried on in to my adult life. It was shortly after having moved into shared accommodation that I woke the entire house up with my screaming. Later, my partner, Liz, experienced the same.

Fortunately, these bouts of screaming nightmares tended to come in fits and starts and people were understanding. They continue to this today. As I write this now at nearly 53 years of age, I had a nightmare last night. Liz was away on business. It was my faithful dog, Rosie, that came up the stairs, jumped on the bed and snuggled me to wake me.

When I had lived alone, the insomnia wasn't such a problem. But when I lived with Liz, I often went to bed much later than her, or would get up in the night to watch TV, read a book, or work.

This started to have an impact on our lives. Liz was getting disturbed by me and not getting sufficient sleep. This caused us to be grumpy and short with each other. We're not prone to arguing, but it was having an effect on our relationship.

The word 'insomnia' had now entered my vocabulary and I learnt it was considered a problem. This caused me to worry about my insomnia. The worry developed into depression.

In my early thirties, I started a new job in the middle of a city centre about twenty-five miles from my home. If I left home to arrive for a 9am start at work, I would have to leave home an hour earlier. If I left home at 7:30am, I would be in for 8am.

The latter was my preference. It meant that I was in the office early and could get lots of work done in a quiet office before most colleagues arrived nearer 9am. Another colleague, Kev, chose to do likewise. Eventually, we became good friends.

One morning when we were alone in the office, I was telling Kev about my insomnia, how I was worried about it, and how it was making me depressed.

'Why are you worried about it?' asked Kev.

'What do you mean?'

'Well, if you miss some sleep you might feel a bit tired or sleepy, but you'll eventually catch up with your sleep again.'

I thought about this. My insomnia began as a child and I had never worried about it as a child because I was unaware it was a 'problem'. Within a week, I stopped worrying about it and simply got on with living.

Please don't be offended by my words if you have insomnia. Insomnia is a condition, like most others, that occurs to varying degrees. For some it is a living hell and I understand and empathise with that.

A very useful book on insomnia is *'An Introduction to Coping with Insomnia and Sleep Problems'* by Colin A. Espie, ISBN 978-1-84901-620-9. The book is recommended by the NHS and the methods it advocates are evidence based. It is widely available, a quick Google will show you where and it is inexpensive.

Chapter 2 – My Snoring

Everybody snores. Probably like most people, I used to only snore occasionally, usually when I was very tired. If I had been drinking, I would snore like a piglet according to Liz. If she was grumpy, because I had badly disturbed her sleep, she would say that I had snored like a pig.

That was fine, or at least tolerable. As people grow older, the trend is for people to get a little heavier. This was the case for me and my snoring got worse. And I snored more often like a pig than a piglet. This was becoming more troublesome.

Then I became chronically ill with ME/CFS. It is an illness that I have written about in many of my books, 'me and my ME' and 'Bear with ME' in particular. ME/CFS has many, many symptoms and fatigue is a primary symptom.

ME/CFS is very difficult to diagnose as no test currently exists for it. Blood tests come up normal. Other chronic illnesses have many common symptoms; fatigue, pain, brain fog, IBS, etc. Consequently, it is difficult to diagnose. It is often misdiagnosed and many medical professionals simply dismiss it as a physiological illness.

But ME/CFS does have a very particular and unusual condition, which can be used to diagnose the condition. For healthy people and even those with chronic illnesses, exercise is good for the health and recovery from illness. This is not the case with ME/CFS.

Post-exertional malaise (PEM) is a considerable worsening of symptoms after even mild physical, mental or emotional activity. This occurs typically one to three days after the activity. PEM can cause a 'crash' where the sufferer is confined to bed until they recover. This can last days, weeks, months or even years in some cases.

It will come as no surprise that people with ME/CFS are desperate to avoid PEM. We do this by pacing ourselves and listening to our bodies. We avoid over exertion, both mental and physical, and try to avoid stress.

So, let's review this. ME/CFS is difficult to diagnose. Diagnosis can take months and frequently years. It's a disease notable for fatigue and is only manageable by rest. When you get it, you know something is wrong with you, but you don't know what it is.

During this period before being diagnosed and learning how to manage your illness, do you think it likely:

A) You would eat normally as you were

B) Eat more

C) Eat less

C is wrong here. Speaking for myself, I ate as normal. Many eat more because they are unhappy with their illness. Regardless, the result is the same. You put on weight because you are fatigued and inactive, and eating more calories than you need.

Over the first two years of having ME/CFS, my weight ballooned. And guess what, I snored like a pig, almost all of the time. This caused Liz to have long-term sleeping problems too.

We began to take turns sleeping in the bedroom, whilst the other slept on the couch downstairs. This is neither good for a relationship, nor you back when you sleep on a couch lots.

The solution seemed to be to turn the spare room, which we used as an office, into a bedroom. This was successful in Liz getting better sleep.

Unfortunately, by now both our backs were in considerable pain from sleeping on the couch for such a long period of time. So, we also had a bespoke couch made to accommodate our specific needs.

The pain in our backs diminished and then went. We were now getting better sleep, but often sleeping apart. And my snoring had got no better. This was an expensive sticking plaster to a big problem, which had not gone away.

Chapter 3 – Sleep Study

But it didn't end there. Things were getting worse. Liz noticed that I seemed to stop breathing during my sleep. This is known as sleep apnea and can be very dangerous both in the short and long-term.

Reluctant at first, Liz persuaded me to go to the GP about my snoring and possible sleep apnea. When I described what you've just read, it was a classic case of symptoms. My GP referred me to a sleep study and it was February.

The sleep study was quite simple. I visited an outpatient clinic in the July and was presented with the study equipment. This is about the size and shape of a large square smart watch, housing electronics and batteries. It also has a flying lead to a finger clip to measure blood oxygen levels and pulse.

After a short lesson on how to use the equipment, I signed the necessary forms. Wearing the study equipment wasn't uncomfortable or bothersome at all.

After a couple of nights wearing the clip and wristband, I returned it to the hospital. It was now August and I was told if there was anything seriously wrong with me, then they would be in touch within a couple of weeks. Otherwise, it could be months before I would hear back from them.

Months passed and I assumed all was well. I considered it unlikely that I had sleep apnea. My snoring hadn't got any better and Liz was growing increasingly concerned about my stopping breathing during my sleep.

In the following February, I had a telephone appointment with a sleep consultant. After asking me several questions, she told me that the data from the sleep study was good quality and a reliable diagnosis could be given. I was diagnosed with insomnia and mild sleep apnea. More specifically, Obstructive Sleep Apnea (OSA).

She offered me a choice of two treatments for the OSA. A mandibular advancement device (MAD) or a Continuous Positive Airway Pressure (CPAP) machine. CPAP is pronounced 'seepap'. Figure 1 shows and example of a MAD and Figure 2 shows a CPAP machine.

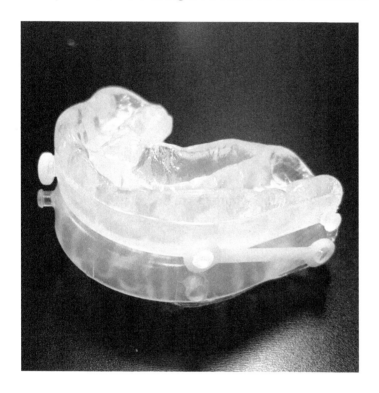

Figure 1. A Mandibular Advancement Device (MAD).

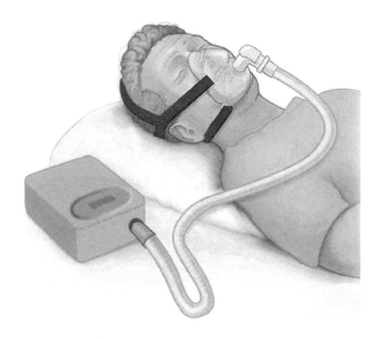

Figure 2. A CPAP machine, hose and face mask.

This was uncharted territory to me, so I had to ask her to explain what these were and I will describe them for you later in this book.

The sleep consultant explained just how dangerous sleep apnea can be. Not treating it because I didn't fancy sleeping with a mouthpiece in or wearing a mask, simply wasn't an option.

Towards the end of the telephone consultation, I was required to choose between a MAD and a CPAP. It was a choice of the lesser of two evils. My experience using a mouthpiece for sports was that it made me gag. Wearing a face mask hooked up to a machine didn't sit well with me either. With a recommendation that the CPAP was usually the more effective treatment, I elected for that.

She then told me that my medical provider was having supply problem difficulties and that I might have to wait about three months to get a CPAP. It had already been a year since I had visited my GP to get a referral. Now, I had a serious medical condition and I had to wait another three months.

This set me thinking. I have a degree in Mechanical Engineering and a PhD in Biomedical Engineering. My earlier investigations had led me to buy and try an anti-snoring mouthpiece. I knew there were lots of inexpensive products available claiming that they cured snoring and sleep apnea.

I had three months until I got my CPAP machine. I was an experienced, highly qualified Bioengineer. Products were available that cost very little. I would buy and test them to see if I could prevent snoring and cure my sleep apnea. What follows in Part Three are my findings.

Part Two
Snoring & Sleep Apnea Explained

Chapter 4 – The Upper Airways

Why do we snore? Snoring is simply vibrations of things such as your throat, mouth, tongue or nasal airways when we breathe during sleep.

Why does it happen? It happens because we relax when we sleep and this causes these parts of the body to narrow. In Figure 3, airflow through the upper airways can be seen for normal sleep and when snoring. You can see how the lower airway has become restricted as the tongue has relaxed and moved towards the throat.

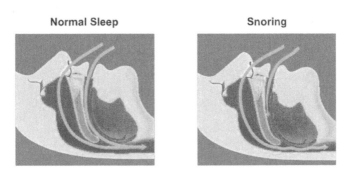

Figure 3: Airflow during sleep and when snoring.

For some people, snoring originates not from the lower airway being obstructed, but the upper nasal airway.

Snoring can also be caused by sleep apnea when the upper airways become temporarily blocked. Figure 4 shows the difference in airflow between snoring and Obstructive Sleep Apnea (OSA). If the upper airway is disrupted causing sleep apnea, it is called Upper Airways Resistance Syndrome (UARS).

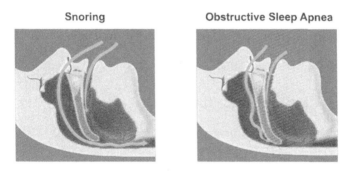

Figure 4: Airflow when snoring and with obstructive sleep apnea.

When OSA occurs, you stop breathing. Fortunately, your brain will always wake you up to restore breathing.

Chapter 5 – Diagnosis

How do we diagnose snoring and sleep apnea?

We know what snoring sounds like, and many of us will have woken ourselves up with our snoring. But it usually your partner who will 'diagnose' your own snoring!

I do not wish to make fun of this. Snoring can be a very serious problem and cause relationship problems. It can even be a major cause in relationship failure.

If you Google, 'snoring test online', you will find a plethora of companies offering free snoring tests. The reason they are free is because after the test, along with your diagnosis their device to cure your snoring will be offered for purchase.

The diagnosis is important because there are different types of snorer. Are you a nose snorer, mouth snorer, tongue snorer or a combination of these? A simple test follows, although more detailed ones are available.

The nose snoring test involves closing one nostril and one's mouth, then attempting to breathe in and out of the other nostril. If the open nostril tends to collapse or close, then you are a nose snorer.

The mouth snoring test begins by inhaling with your mouth open, mimicking the typical snoring noise. Next, repeat this but with your mouth closed. If you cannot replicate the snoring sound, you are probably a mouth snorer.

The throat snorer test begins like the mouth snoring test. Inhale with your mouth open, mimicking the typical snoring noise. Next, repeat this but with your tongue sticking out, gently clamped by your teeth. If you cannot replicate the snoring sound, you are probably a throat snorer.

What sort of snorer are you? This will help you choose which anti-snoring products might be applicable to you. And crucially, which will likely be of no use to you.

Sleep apnea should be diagnosed by an appropriate medical professional via a sleep study. However, you can make a tentative diagnosis yourself, particularly with help from your partner. If you live alone and are concerned that you may have sleep apnea, you could make a recording of you sleeping to see if any of the following symptoms are evident:

- Breathing stopping and starting
- Waking up frequently
- Loud snoring
- Making snorting, gasping or choking noises.

It is not just when you are asleep that you may notice problems from sleep apnea. You may wake up with a headache. During the day you might feel the following:

- Tired and fatigued
- Have difficulty concentrating
- Have mood swings
- Prone to falling asleep during the day

If you have any of the major symptoms, you should see your GP. Taking your partner with you to describe the symptoms they have observed may be helpful.

Sleep apnea can be dangerous if it is not diagnosed and treated. Left untreated, sleep apnea can cause high blood pressure, diabetes, heart diseases, depression and give you a higher chance of having a stroke.

Other dangers with sleep apnea should be obvious. If you are having difficulty concentrating and sometimes fall asleep, operating machinery or driving a vehicle are clearly dangerous.

The National Health Service (NHS) website states,

'If sleep apnea has been confirmed, you must not drive until your symptoms are under control.'

However, a check of the Driving Vehicle and Licensing Agency (DVLA) website will show that this is not strictly true. The DVLA website says,

'You must not drive until you're free from excessive sleepiness or until your symptoms are under control and you're strictly following any necessary treatment.'

I am not splitting hairs here. It is quite possible to have sleep apnea and not be excessively sleepy. By following the NHS advice rather than the DVLA advice could impact on your job, caring for people, etc. if you were to unnecessarily stop driving.

Please be very clear though, I am not advocating driving if your condition would render driving to be dangerous.

You must tell DVLA if you have:

- *confirmed moderate or severe obstructive sleep apnea syndrome (OSAS), with excessive sleepiness*
- *either narcolepsy or cataplexy, or both*
- *any other sleep condition that has caused excessive sleepiness for at least 3 months - including suspected or confirmed mild OSAS*

Chapter 6 – Treatments

Snoring is much more likely if you are overweight, smoke, drink too much alcohol or sleep on your back. It's not something you can stop at will, neither can it be cured. But snoring can be treated and there are several things you can do yourself to help treat your snoring.

- Try losing weight if you are overweight
- Sleep on your side
- Stop smoking
- Do not drink too much alcohol
- Do not take sleeping pills

How to do most of these things should be obvious. If you want to know how to lose weight, there are many ways to do this and this book isn't a diet book. Look elsewhere.

But how to sleep on your side? There are several ways to do this. You can use pillows to prop you up. Special pillows and bed wedges can be bought to do this. Personally, I've never enjoyed much success with these.

You can also either buy an anti-snoring vest, or make something to do the same yourself. The gist of this solution is to wear something in the middle of your back, which is uncomfortable to lie on. You will naturally turn on to your side to avoid the discomfort.

As I snore on my back, side and front, upside down and probably under water too, this latter solution isn't an option for me. Fortunately, other solutions are available.

As we have learnt, snoring and the more serious condition, sleep apnea, are caused by narrowing or even blocking of the upper airways. Most anti-snoring and sleep apnea devices attempt, or rather supposedly attempt, to keep these airways open.

In the next section of the book, you will read about my experiences and experiments with several of these devices. In the meantime, let us consider the two solutions available on the NHS.

Chapter 7 – Mandibular Advancement Device

A mandibular advancement device (MAD) is a type of mouthpiece. It should be made by an appropriately qualified dentist. We saw an example of a MAD in Figure 1 and another is shown below in Figure 5.

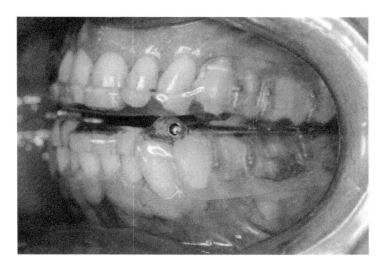

Figure 5. A Mandibular Advancement Device (MAD).

A MAD is intended to move the lower jaw forward. In doing so, it also moves the tongue forward and it helps to keep the airways open to prevent snoring and sleep apnea.

These devices can help with other conditions of the teeth too, such as teeth grinding.

There are potential drawbacks to using a MAD. They can be uncomfortable to wear and cause aching of the teeth, gums and jaw. They can also lead to an excessive production of saliva as the brain thinks you are eating. This can lead to dribbling.

Long-term use of a MAD can cause other problems such as teeth loosening. Gum problems are also possible such as bleeding and recession. It can also cause arthritis in the joint of the jaw.

Clearly, we need another treatment. And we have one, CPAP.

The gold standard treatment for sleep apnea is a CPAP machine. We saw a drawing of a CPAP in Figure 2 and a picture of one is shown below in Figure 6.

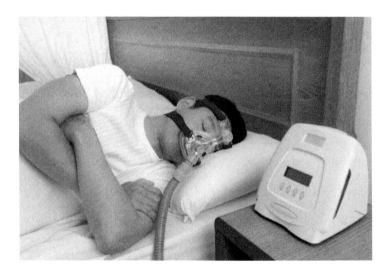

Figure 6. A CPAP machine connected to a face mask via a hose.

A CPAP provides a positive air pressure, delivered from the machine via a tube to a mask worn on the face. The positive pressure keeps the upper airways open and prevents OSA.

The positive pressure keeps the airways open and improves quality of sleep. Studies have shown that for some people it can reduce both high blood pressure and reduce the risk of stroke.

Understandably, wearing a facemask connected to a machine via a hose, doesn't come naturally when you are trying to sleep. It can take weeks, even months to get used to wearing a CPAP. Perseverance is required. Remember, this thing is very likely extending your life and possibly saving you from a very early departure.

You will be given help by a suitably trained person on how to fit the mask and set the machine up for your requirements. Regular cleaning of various parts of the CPAP are also required, which you will be shown. There are several sleep apnea groups on Facebook, which you may find useful. However, as ever follow the advice of your GP or Consultant.

There are other considerations to life with CPAP. For example, the need to take it with you when you go on holiday or away overnight with work. Smaller travel

CPAP's are available, but they are power hungry devices so you will need to fully consider how you will power one.

CPAP's are not only power hungry, they are also expensive. By expensive, I mean hundreds of dollars, pounds or more, depending on your currency.

If you look online, you will see many mini- or micro-CPAP's for sale. These are small devices which sit on your nose and contain a small rechargeable battery. Could they possibly work? In Part Three we will take a light-hearted look at several anti-snoring and sleep apnea devices.

Part Three

Device Experiments

Chapter 9 – Explanation and Experiments

It is worth mentioning a little about myself before we discuss experiments. I'm not some crank testing products willy-nilly. I have many years industrial experience as an Engineer and I have a degree in Mechanical Engineering. More than that, I have a PhD in Biomedical Engineering with a career spanning over two and a half decades.

I have taken a look at several products commonly available to purchase online. In the following pages, I will discuss each device in turn looking at:

- What they claim to do
- Any possible reasons that they may work
- Results of my testing them in various ways
- Whether they are worth buying

You will see in the tests that whenever an item contained any electronics, I broke out the tools to investigate further. For all the devices I tested, I had three ways of evaluating their success.

I had my own experiences of wearing and using each device. I also had the trusty Liz to confirm, or otherwise, a cessation or reduction in my snoring, snorting and other guttural utterances.

What I also had, was a smart watch. Smart watches, smart rings and other wearable telemetry are widely available to monitor your sleep. Typically, these measure heart rate and blood oxygen levels.

Algorithms then analyse the data and can offer up analysis of your sleep quality, length of REM and other sleep phases. Some will crucially provide you with the frequency of sleep apnea episodes.

But which device do I recommend, I hear you ask? Within a month of writing my recommendation down, it will be usurped by another new product. But not to leave you at a loss as to which one to buy, you will not go far wrong buying from established smart watch brands. Do a bit of research. There are lots of articles online to read or watch on YouTube.

What you need to do is wear the smart product for at least a few days to establish your baseline. Then, if you try an anti-snoring or sleep apnea device, you will get data from your smart device to compare with your baseline. This will tell you if things have improved or not, and by how much.

A CPAP machine comes suitably equipped to collect such data. This then allows the machine to be fine-tuned perfectly for you.

What I must say is that these are my personal findings. Another person might get a different result due to the reasons for their own snoring or sleep apnea. Nevertheless, some results are applicable to everybody.

Now, let the fun begin! In this Section I test the miracle products available online, typically costing no more than a few pounds or dollars!

Chapter 10 – Mouthpieces

Any online search for 'anti-snoring devices', 'sleep apnea devices' or 'snoring aids' will produce a variety of mouthpieces. You will find the same products when you search for 'teeth grinding guards' or 'sports mouth guards'.

These inexpensive devices, whatever they claim to be, are not the same as a MAD made by a qualified dental technician or dentist, costing hundreds of dollars or pounds.

In Figure 7, you can see the very mouth piece that I bought and used. Such devices usually claim to stop snoring and prevent sleep apnea. Many erroneously claim to be recommended by the NHS or other medical provider.

Could they work? Well, you're familiar with MAD's now, which are recommended, and push the jaw forward to keep airways open

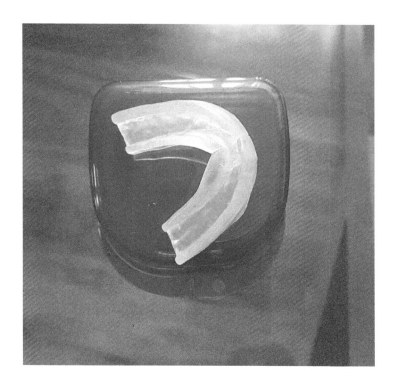

Figure 7. Mouthpiece sat on the box to store it in.

I suspect these inexpensive devices were designed as either cheap sports mouth guards or teeth grinding guards. Most people have neither an overbite nor an underbite and will therefore hold the jaw in a fairly neutral position. This then fails to achieve the main purpose of a MAD, advancing the jaw.

If you had an overbite, then they would have a chance or working as a MAD by advancing the lower jaw. By contrast, if you had an underbite then the device would actually make the situation worse.

By and large, these products typically claim to be made of a medical grade plastic and come with instructions for use. You are required to boil some water then dunk the device in the water for a short period. You then need to remove it from the water without scolding yourself, quickly pop it into your mouth and then bite down. After another short period, you then dunk the mouthpiece in cold water to set the impression of your teeth.

The actual instructions that came with my device, I followed exactly. To do this I used both a stopwatch and a temperature probe. After the first attempt, it had a fairly rudimentary impression of my teeth and didn't sit well in my mouth. So, I repeated the exercise. Second time round, the mouthpiece fitted rather well.

Some of the factors I have already written about for MAD's proved accurate with this mouthpiece. And not in a good way. I drooled like a dog watching someone eating a chocolate bar. My teeth, gums and jaw ached.

Another problem I found was that the mouthpiece would usually fall out during the night. Upon waking in the dark of the middle of the night, I was usually unable to locate it to pop it back in.

But I did find that I slept better with it and Liz confirmed a reduction in my snoring volume. After a few days of wearing it, I probably grew conditioned to having it in my mouth and it would go AWOL less frequently. On a morning, my mouth was not dry and my throat not sore as they were prior to testing.

Why did it seem to work to some extent for me? It was because I was sleeping more with my mouth closed and breathing through my nose. I do not have a problem with my nasal airway.

Would I recommend it? These might work for throat and mouth snorers. If you have an underbite, they be more applicable to you. My thoughts are that you should probably only try these if some other products you have tried have failed to help you.

Chapter 11 – Micro-CPAP

I will admit at the very start that I knew as an Engineer, that the various mini- and micro-CPAP devices sold inexpensively online, would not work. The reasons for this are several. These devices vents to atmosphere so cannot generate a positive pressure, the very essence of what they are supposed to do.

Also, the energy requirements of a suitable fan would determine a battery size which could not possibly fit in a device of such a small size. However, battery design is progressing quickly and it is not inconceivable that a mini-CPAP machine could be viable within a few years. Obviously, such a machine would look nothing like these pieces of tat. And with that, I refer you to Figure 8 and the micro-CPAP that I bought and tested.

I will continue with my annihilation of this useless device that I purchased. If the mouthpiece that I had previously tested would go AWOL occasionally, this thing wouldn't even stay in position on my nose long enough to get the chance to go AWOL. Hopeless!

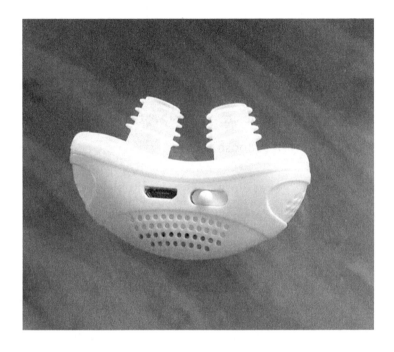

Figure 8. A micro-CPAP.

Once fully charged and turned on, I could feel the smallest of vibrations hinting at the two fans within it turning. These can be seen by looking through the nostril fixtures, which don't fixate!

The small vibrations that I could feel were smaller than the air flow that I couldn't feel from the device. I began by trying to see just how ludicrously small this breeze was by trying to blow pieces of paper, plastic and hairs.

Nothing moved, so I resorted to attempting to blow bubbles. As you can see in Figure 9, I smeared a film of soapy water across both nasal exhaust protrusions.

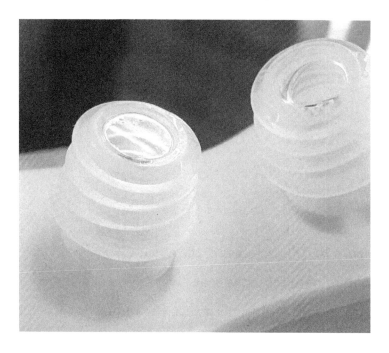

Figure 9. Soapy water covering the nasal exhausts of the micro-CPAP with the device turned off.

It was with much glee and laughter when I observed what happened to the soapy films when I turned the device on. You can make out in Figure 10, more so on the left-hand side nasal exhaust, that all that happened was that the film began to show swirling patterns.

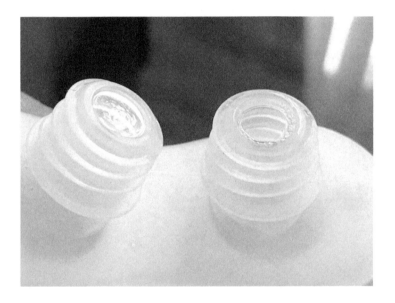

Figure 10. The twin fans of the micro-CPAP caused swirling patterns in the soapy water films across the nasal exhausts when the device was turned on.

I was really enjoying myself so I now took the device apart. In Figure 11, you can see what I found.

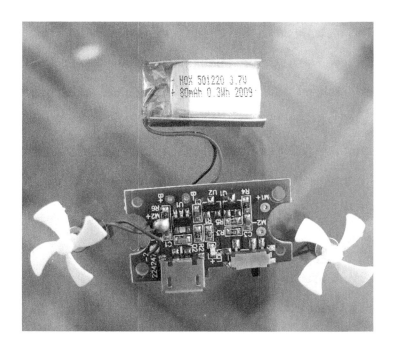

Figure 11. The inner workings of the micro-CPAP.

You can see it has two small fans with their own individual tiny motors. It has a small circuit board that looks to be manufactured well. Indeed, the entire device is manufactured to a decent standard. Shame it doesn't work.

You can also see to the top of Figure 11, a small rechargeable battery. It has writing on it, such as '3.7V', '80mAh' and '0.3Wh'. It also has '2009' written on it.

This indicates that the battery was manufactured some fourteen years before I bought it. The device was probably made around the same time and has sat in a warehouse all that time. To be fair, when I fully charged the battery, I measured a healthy 4.1 Volts across the battery terminals, rather more than the specified 3.7 Volts.

After measuring a few more things and calculating just how long this battery would keep those fans running, I put it back together. After fully charging it, I turned it on and set my stopwatch running to see just how long it would run for.

It was running at 3 hrs 15 minutes, but had stopped by 3 hrs 30 minutes. Please excuse my tardiness at witnessing the very second the fans stopped turning. Even if it worked, which it doesn't, it failed to run for the minimum period of 4 hours that a CPAP should be used every night.

Do I need to tell you whether this thing is worth buying? Probably not, but I'll do it anyway. If you have ever looked at one of these and wondered about giving it a go, it's only ten bucks, then don't wonder anymore. It's a complete waste of money.

Unless of course you're a nerdy Engineer like me. I got every penny worth of value out of testing it.

I'm not a nose snorer, but in the interests of testing, I ordered what the advert described as a 'Highly Recommended' magnetic nose clip. It is shown in Figure 12.

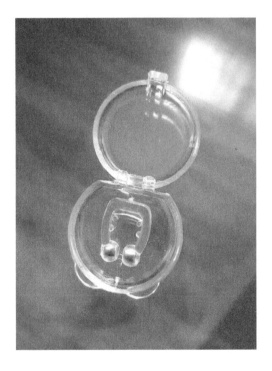

Figure 12. The 'Highly Recommended' magnetic nose clip.

According to the adverts, these are supposedly effective, fit perfectly, are easy to use, reliably secure, and made of medical silicone and BPA (bisphenol A) free.

In Figure 13, you can see how one goes about inserting them into your nose, so that they 'fit perfectly'.

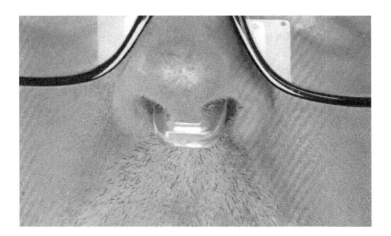

Figure 13. Magnetic nose clips 'fit perfectly'.

There are some people who suffer from a deviated septum. This is a condition where the septum, the thin wall that separates your nasal cavities, is displaced to one side. This can result in only one nostril working effectively. For such a person, this clip may help them.

For most other snoring issues, the magnetic nose clip is unlikely to offer little benefit. Having said that, I personally found it mildly uncomfortable and the presence of it caused me to flair my nostrils slightly. For a nose snorer with a similar reaction to me, the faint hope of this device working is there. However, when you sleep your body relaxes and I very much doubt that these would then cause nasal flaring.

In summary, unless you have a deviated septum avoid them. And if you have a deviated septum, make a GP appointment and get appropriate medical advice. Enough said.

Chapter 13 – Nasal Dilators

Keeping with the nasal device theme, I ordered a pack of nasal dilators. Figure 14 shows a nasal dilator and the storage box for them.

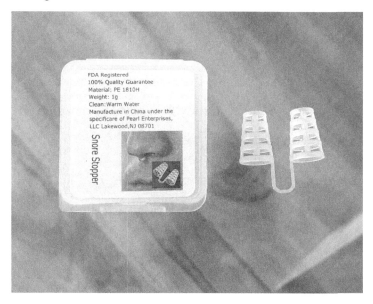

Figure 14. Nasal dilator and storage box.

They are supposed to do what they say, dilate the nasal passages. They look like they may indeed do this. If you are a nose snorer and your snoring originates from your nasal passages, I think that they have a decent chance of working. If your snoring originates further along the upper airway, for example in upper nasal cavity, then they are unlikely to offer much help.

I didn't find these uncomfortable and they sat rather snugly in my nose. They did stay in place all night and didn't make a bid for freedom and go AWOL like some other products.

I'm not a nose snorer, so they were unlikely to reduce or stop my snoring. And they didn't. That's not to say, they wouldn't work for a nose snorer.

For a nose snorer, as these cost buttons, I would recommend giving them a try. Thumbs up from Bear!

Chapter 14 – Smart Throat Snorer Stopper

Next a product for throat snorers, the 'Smart Throat Snorer', as shown in Figure 15.

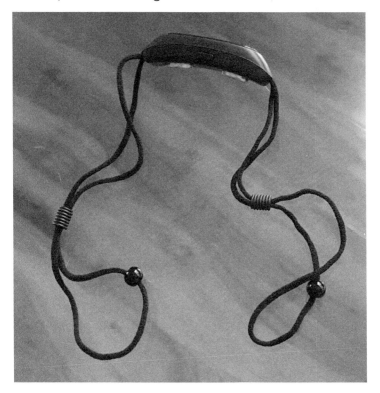

Figure 15. Smart (really?) throat snorer stopper.

These are held against the skin in the area of the throat, by two loops of elastic which pass behind your ears. On the side touching your skin are two metal pads. On the outer side are six, blue LED lights.

The adverts say that the device can detect snoring, *'through high-precision sensors'*. No description of how this works is offered. For example, do they audibly detect snoring, is it by vibration or some other way?

They then claim to *'massage the hypoglossal nerve and mandibular muscle with different frequency vibration pulse to promote muscle tightening'*. This apparently adjusts breathing rhythm to make breathing smoother, with a *'significant anti-snoring effect'*.

Could snoring be detected through an unspecified *'high-precision'* sensor? As an Engineer, I would have thought it highly possible to detect snoring with a suitable sensor and algorithm. The problem for me here is that for the device to be effective, you want to detect the indications that snoring is about to start so that you can prevent snoring happening.

Could the device do what it claims? It is a possibility.

And so, to testing. As ever, I followed the instructions provided by the manufacturer. As with almost every product tested, none came with this device. So, I followed the words and pictures in the advert.

What I discovered was that I could not feel anything massaging my throat. My snoring was reduced in volume a little. My mouth wasn't dry in the morning or my throat sore, indicating that I hadn't been breathing through my mouth. I put this down to the device and the elastic loops over my ears, being fairly effective at keeping my mouth closed when I slept.

I did less sleeping wearing this device than I would have liked. Why, I hear you ask? The six blue LED lights on the device, that's why. I felt like I had a blue torch held under my chin. The light really interrupted my sleep.

It was so noticeable, that I looked round my bedroom to see what other lights were there that didn't normally disrupt my sleep. There four other sources of light, all red and dimly lit, indicating devices were powered and on standby. The contrast with the six blue lights strapped to my chin was remarkable.

Following real world sleep testing, I broke out the tools again and opened up the smart throat snorer stopper, which you can see in Figure 16.

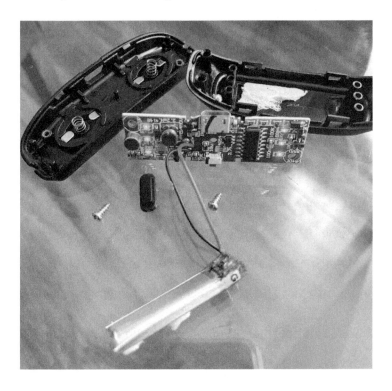

Figure 16. The innards of the smart throat snorer stopper.

What you get the sense of in Figure 15 is the brightness of the six blue LED's. The picture was taken in a brightly lit room. Even in a well-lit room, you can clearly see from the picture just how intense the light from the blue LED's is. Imagine that in the dark, when you are trying to sleep. It makes me tired thinking about it.

The metal pads that pressed against the throat did not move and were connected to the device each by a spring. No mechanism existed in the device to generate a vibration, which wouldn't have worked anyway.

Over various tests I could only detect the faintest of electrical potential across the two metal pads, insufficient to have any effect on an adult. Or a baby. Or a baby mouse. Or possibly anything.

Just in case I was missing anything here, I decided to see how long the device would run for on a single charge. If the device was massaging *'the hypoglossal nerve and mandibular muscle with different frequency vibration pulse to promote muscle tightening'* it would use energy to do so. Hopefully, the rechargeable battery in the snorer would keep the lights and the massaging mechanism going for eight hours of good sleep.

The test became a marathon. The battery eventually ran out of charge after nearly forty hours. That's nearly five nights, each of eight hours sleep. If the mechanism was working, it would be using energy and the battery would have stopped much earlier. It's a little surprising that the little rechargeable battery powered six LED's for nearly forty hours.

Would I recommend buying one? No, I would not. However, what did surprise me how effective the device was at diminishing snoring by virtue of holding my mouth closed with two pieces of elastic. This prompted me to choose the next device to test.

Chapter 15 – Anti-Snoring Chin Strap

The anti-snoring chin strap is essentially a neoprene belt that passes under the chin and over the head to hold the mouth shut. You can see one in Figure 17.

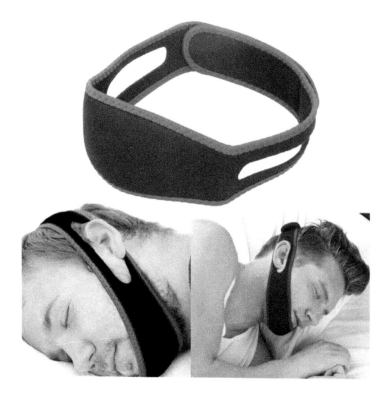

Figure 17. The anti-snoring chin strap.

Cheap and simple, the strap uses Velcro to accommodate different head sizes. The same also serves to adjust the tightness of the strap. Along both sides of the strap are oblong holes, which the pictures in the advert indicate are for your ears to pass through.

Presumably, the device is designed to hold the mouth closed during sleeping and prevent snoring. This is plausible.

However, if you look at Figure 16 again, you will see that the two male models are wearing the strap in different ways. On the left, the strap is under the chin holding the mouth closed. On the right, the strap is over the chin, holding the mouth closed and pushing the jaw back. This is the very opposite of what the science tells us what we want – remember the mandibular advancement device (MAD).

Nevertheless, I found the device did reduce my snoring volume and it was comfortable to wear. After the first night, I had to tighten the strap as the neoprene had likely stretched a little. It was a little difficult to adjust the tension of the strap to ensure the mouth was held shut, without the strap being uncomfortably tight.

This set me thinking and I will be making my own prototype snoring device. The first prototype did reduce my snoring further and led me think of an evolution of the design. Perhaps more on a new snoring aid in the future….

Would I recommend the neoprene one you can buy now? If you are a mouth or throat snorer, I would suggest giving it a go. It's one of the cheapest products I tested, it was comfortable and diminished my snoring. Depending on the severity of your snoring problem, it may help.

Chapter 16 – Anti-Snoring Tongue Device

And finally, the anti-snoring tongue device, as shown in Figure 18.

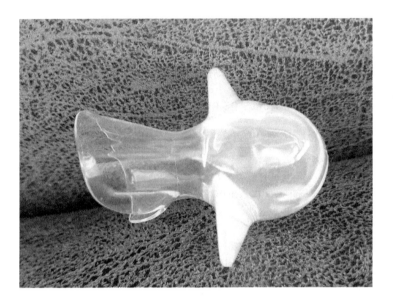

Figure 18. The anti-snoring tongue device.

This device is intended to hold the tip of your tongue by vacuum in a bulb, on the right of this image, protruding from your mouth. This will then move the back of the tongue forward, opening the airway and preventing snoring.

The 'fins' in the middle of the product sit outside your lips and prevent the device moving back into your mouth.

The concept is rather novel compared with all other devices I have seen and tested. Theoretically, it actually has a chance of working.

Unfortunately, it didn't work for me. If I forced my tongue as far into the bulb as possible, it caused me to wretch. Sorry. If I positioned my tongue at a comfortable / bearable extension then before long the 'vacuum' would be broken and the device would fall from my mouth.

I also had a fear that if I fell asleep with my tongue out, my teeth might clasp my tongue and bite it off!

Verdict, not for me. If you are comfortable with your tongue extended from your mouth for eight hours and don't expect to bite your own tongue off, then perhaps you might be interested. Good luck with that!

Part Four

Conclusions

Chapter 17 – Conclusions

Snoring is very serious and can damage, even destroy relationships. To prevent that happening, we need to do something about snoring. Sleeping in another room, may be a solution for some. However, for many couples sharing the marital bed is extremely important to them. So, we need to address snoring another way.

In Chapter 5 we discussed how to diagnose different types of snoring. This is important in determining whether you are a nose, mouth, throat or combination of these type snorer. Armed with that knowledge, you can then choose an appropriate anti-snoring device.

For nose snorers, the nasal dilators that were tested are recommended. Whether these are successful, will depend on the origin of the nose snoring, for example in the lower nasal cavity versus the upper. However, they are inexpensive, readily available, comfortable and simple to use. Why not give them ago?

For mouth and throat snorers, the anti-snoring chin strap is inexpensive, comfortable, possibly will dimmish snoring to some extent but maybe not stop it.

If you are a mouth snorer with an underbite, then one of the inexpensive mouthpiece devices is perhaps worth trying. However, these aren't device made precisely to fit your own mouth by a suitably trained professional. Teeth loosening, gum problems and long-term the potential of arthritis in the jaw joint, dissuade me from long-term use with such a generic product.

The rest of the products are quite frankly, a waste of money. For many people with snoring or sleep apnea problems, they can help their situation by losing weight, stopping smoking, cutting back on alcohol, avoiding sleeping pills and sleeping on their side.

Sleep apnea can be very dangerous if untreated. In Chapter 5 we discussed some typical symptoms of sleep apnea. If you identify with any of these, you should contact your GP. If you suspect or are concerned that you may have sleep apnea, you must seek medical advice. Diagnosis of sleep apnea should be by a suitably qualified medical professional using a sleep study.

Clinically tested and proven treatment of sleep apnea is by either a Mandibular Advancement Device (MAD), or CPAP machine. These are discussed in Chapters 7 and 8 respectively. CPAP is the gold standard treatment for sleep apnea, but requires perseverance to use and tolerate.

Thank you for reading. You may enjoy other books in the Bear the Awarenessist series.

Bear with ME is a collection of humorous, heart-warming and heart-breaking articles and stories about Long Covid, Fibromyalgia, ME/CFS and other chronic illnesses.

Bear in Mind reveals the true stores of the bullying Bear endured at school, university and at work. If you poke the Bear, you should expect him to react!

Printed in Great Britain
by Amazon

23746469R00046